After months of waiting, Congratulations! It's such an exciting time, but for most new parents, it can also be a bit overwhelming. All of the unknowns and intricacies of every day can become a blur. And while chances are you'll be thrilled, there's also a good chance you'll have questions–lots and lots of questions... Is the baby eating enough? How much sleep should the baby be getting? Is poop supposed to be yellow? Recording all of your baby's daily activities enables you to track their development and recognize your baby's natural schedule. Plus, this information becomes an important tool in providing your pediatrician with the details needed to help evaluate your baby's general health and development.

The Baby's Eat, Sleep & Poop Journal® - A baby's life and daily log book was truly born out of necessity. As new and clueless parents, the small effort of writing down our baby's daily routine had big results. It was so reassuring and really helped us to be sure our daughter was meeting all of her nutritional requirements and progressing normally. Many hospitals and pediatricians recommend documenting this information–everyone I knew was using loose scraps of paper or notebooks. I realized I wasn't the only sleep-deprived mom who needed this kind of record-keeper... So, we developed this all-inclusive, easy-to-use journal to capture and organize this valuable information and help new parents, like you, be sure your baby is healthy & happy.

If you have any questions or comments, feel free to email us at:
info@eatsleeppoop.com or visit **EatSleepPoop.com**

Best to you & baby!
Sandra Kosak

The Baby's Eat, Sleep & Poop Journal® is printed in the USA and is a registered trademark. ©2004-2020. Without limiting the rights under copyright reserved, no part of this publication may be reproduced or transmitted in any form, by any means without the written consent of the author. The scanning, uploading and distribution of this book via the internet is illegal and punishable by law.

Notes & Milestones:

This Baby's Eat, Sleep & Poop Journal® belongs to:

_____

Important Names & Numbers

Pediatrician: _____

Pediatrician's Emergency Service: _____

Lactation Specialist: _____

OB/GYN: _____

Insurance: _____

Hospital: _____

Other: _____

_____

_____

Emergency: 911   Poison Control: 1(800) 222-1222

For more information visit EatSleepPoop.com

©2004-2020 SK Creative Agency Inc. All rights reserved. eatsleeppoop.com

Notes & Milestones:

Baby's Growth Chart & Immunization Record

Birthday: _____ Blood Type: _____

Date	Weight & Percentile			Length & Percentile		Head & Percentile	
	lbs.	oz.	%	in.	%	in.	%
	lbs.	oz.	%	in.	%	in.	%
	lbs.	oz.	%	in.	%	in.	%
	lbs.	oz.	%	in.	%	in.	%
	lbs.	oz.	%	in.	%	in.	%
	lbs.	oz.	%	in.	%	in.	%
	lbs.	oz.	%	in.	%	in.	%
	lbs.	oz.	%	in.	%	in.	%
	lbs.	oz.	%	in.	%	in.	%
	lbs.	oz.	%	in.	%	in.	%

Vaccines	Dates				
Hepatitis B	1:	2:	3:		
Diphtheria, Tetanus, & Pertussis	1:	2:	3:	4:	5:
H. Influenza Type B	1:	2:	3:	4:	
Polio	1:	2:	3:	4:	
Pneumococcal	1:	2:	3:	4:	5:
Rotavirus	1:	2:	3:		
Measles, Mumps & Rubella	1:	2:			
Varicella	1:	2:			
Influenza	1:	2:	3:	4:	5:
Hepatitis A	1:	2:			

Notes & Milestones:

Baby's Icky-Sicky Record

Date	Doctor & Diagnosis	Medication & Dosage (& Breastfeeding, Mom's Medication)

Medical Conditions _____

Allergies _____

Other _____

_____

Notes & Milestones:

Baby's Eat, Sleep & Poop Daily Activity

DATE	TIME	MINUTES (Breastfeeding)	OUNCES (Bottle)	SLEEP / WAKE	WET	POOP
		LEFT:				
		RIGHT:				
		L:				
		R:				
		L:				
		R:				
		L:				
		R:				
		L:				
		R:				
		L:				
		R:				
		L:				
		R:				
		L:				
		R:				
		L:				
		R:				
		L:				
		R:				
		L:				
		R:				
		L:				
		R:				
		L:				
		R:				

©2004-2020 SK Creative Agency Inc. All rights reserved. eatsleeppoop.com

Notes & Milestones:

Baby's Eat, Sleep & Poop Daily Activity

DATE	TIME	MINUTES (Breastfeeding)	OUNCES (Bottle)	SLEEP WAKE	WET	POOP
		LEFT				
		RIGHT				
		L:				
		R:				
		L:				
		R:				
		L:				
		R:				
		L:				
		R:				
		L:				
		R:				
		L:				
		R:				
		L:				
		R:				
		L:				
		R:				
		L:				
		R:				
		L:				
		R:				
		L:				
		R:				
		L:				
		R:				

©2004-2020 SK Creative Agency Inc. All rights reserved. eatsleeppoop.com

Notes & Milestones:

Baby's Eat, Sleep & Poop Daily Activity

DATE	TIME	MINUTES (Breastfeeding)	OUNCES (Bottle)	SLEEP / WAKE	WET	POOP
		LEFT				
		RIGHT				
		L:				
		R:				
		L:				
		R:				
		L:				
		R:				
		L:				
		R:				
		L:				
		R:				
		L:				
		R:				
		L:				
		R:				
		L:				
		R:				
		L:				
		R:				
		L:				
		R:				
		L:				
		R:				
		L:				
		R:				

©2004-2020 SK Creative Agency Inc. All rights reserved. eatsleeppoop.com

Notes & Milestones:

Baby's Eat, Sleep & Poop Daily Activity

DATE	TIME	MINUTES (Breastfeeding)	OUNCES (Bottle)	SLEEP / WAKE	WET	POOP
		LEFT				
		RIGHT				
		L:				
		R:				
		L:				
		R:				
		L:				
		R:				
		L:				
		R:				
		L:				
		R:				
		L:				
		R:				
		L:				
		R:				
		L:				
		R:				
		L:				
		R:				
		L:				
		R:				
		L:				
		R:				
		L:				
		R:				

©2004-2020 SK Creative Agency Inc. All rights reserved. eatsleeppoop.com

Notes & Milestones:

Baby's Eat, Sleep & Poop Daily Activity

DATE	TIME	MINUTES (Breastfeeding)	OUNCES (Bottle)	SLEEP WAKE	WET	POOP
		LEFT				
		RIGHT				
		L:				
		R:				
		L:				
		R:				
		L:				
		R:				
		L:				
		R:				
		L:				
		R:				
		L:				
		R:				
		L:				
		R:				
		L:				
		R:				
		L:				
		R:				
		L:				
		R:				
		L:				
		R:				
		L:				
		R:				

©2004-2020 SK Creative Agency Inc. All rights reserved. eatsleeppoop.com

Notes & Milestones:

Baby's Eat, Sleep & Poop Daily Activity

DATE	TIME	MINUTES (Breastfeeding)	OUNCES (Bottle)	SLEEP / WAKE	WET	POOP
		LEFT				
		RIGHT				
		L:				
		R:				
		L:				
		R:				
		L:				
		R:				
		L:				
		R:				
		L:				
		R:				
		L:				
		R:				
		L:				
		R:				
		L:				
		R:				
		L:				
		R:				
		L:				
		R:				
		L:				
		R:				
		L:				
		R:				

Notes & Milestones:

Baby's Eat, Sleep & Poop Daily Activity

DATE	TIME	MINUTES (Breastfeeding)	OUNCES (Bottle)	SLEEP / WAKE	WET	POOP
		LEFT				
		RIGHT				
		L:				
		R:				
		L:				
		R:				
		L:				
		R:				
		L:				
		R:				
		L:				
		R:				
		L:				
		R:				
		L:				
		R:				
		L:				
		R:				
		L:				
		R:				
		L:				
		R:				
		L:				
		R:				
		L:				
		R:				

©2004-2020 SK Creative Agency Inc. All rights reserved. eatsleeppoop.com

Notes & Milestones:

Baby's Eat, Sleep & Poop Daily Activity

DATE	TIME	MINUTES (Breastfeeding)	OUNCES (Bottle)	SLEEP / WAKE	WET	POOP
		LEFT				
		RIGHT				
		L:				
		R:				
		L:				
		R:				
		L:				
		R:				
		L:				
		R:				
		L:				
		R:				
		L:				
		R:				
		L:				
		R:				
		L:				
		R:				
		L:				
		R:				
		L:				
		R:				
		L:				
		R:				
		L:				
		R:				

Notes & Milestones:

Baby's Eat, Sleep & Poop Daily Activity

DATE	TIME	MINUTES (Breastfeeding)	OUNCES (Bottle)	SLEEP / WAKE	WET	POOP
		LEFT:				
		RIGHT:				
		L:				
		R:				
		L:				
		R:				
		L:				
		R:				
		L:				
		R:				
		L:				
		R:				
		L:				
		R:				
		L:				
		R:				
		L:				
		R:				
		L:				
		R:				
		L:				
		R:				
		L:				
		R:				
		L:				
		R:				

Notes & Milestones:

Baby's Eat, Sleep & Poop Daily Activity

DATE	TIME	MINUTES (Breastfeeding)	OUNCES (Bottle)	SLEEP / WAKE	WET	POOP
		LEFT				
		RIGHT				
		L:				
		R:				
		L:				
		R:				
		L:				
		R:				
		L:				
		R:				
		L:				
		R:				
		L:				
		R:				
		L:				
		R:				
		L:				
		R:				
		L:				
		R:				
		L:				
		R:				
		L:				
		R:				
		L:				
		R:				

©2004-2020 SK Creative Agency Inc. All rights reserved. eatsleeppoop.com

Notes & Milestones:

Baby's Eat, Sleep & Poop Daily Activity

DATE	TIME	MINUTES (Breastfeeding)		OUNCES (Bottle)	SLEEP WAKE	WET	POOP
		LEFT					
		RIGHT					
		L:					
		R:					
		L:					
		R:					
		L:					
		R:					
		L:					
		R:					
		L:					
		R:					
		L:					
		R:					
		L:					
		R:					
		L:					
		R:					
		L:					
		R:					
		L:					
		R:					
		L:					
		R:					
		L:					
		R:					

©2004-2020 SJK Creative Agency Inc. All rights reserved. eatsleeppoop.com

Notes & Milestones:

Baby's Eat, Sleep & Poop Daily Activity

DATE	TIME	MINUTES (Breastfeeding)	OUNCES (Bottle)	SLEEP WAKE	WET	POOP
		LEFT				
		RIGHT				
		L:				
		R:				
		L:				
		R:				
		L:				
		R:				
		L:				
		R:				
		L:				
		R:				
		L:				
		R:				
		L:				
		R:				
		L:				
		R:				
		L:				
		R:				
		L:				
		R:				
		L:				
		R:				
		L:				
		R:				

©2004-2020 SK Creative Agency Inc. All rights reserved. eatsleeppoop.com

Notes & Milestones:

Baby's Eat, Sleep & Poop Daily Activity

DATE	TIME	MINUTES (Breastfeeding)	OUNCES (Bottle)	SLEEP WAKE	WET	POOP
		LEFT				
		RIGHT				
		L:				
		R:				
		L:				
		R:				
		L:				
		R:				
		L:				
		R:				
		L:				
		R:				
		L:				
		R:				
		L:				
		R:				
		L:				
		R:				
		L:				
		R:				
		L:				
		R:				
		L:				
		R:				
		L:				
		R:				
		L:				
		R:				

Notes & Milestones:

Baby's Eat, Sleep & Poop Daily Activity

DATE	TIME	MINUTES (Breastfeeding)	OUNCES (Bottle)	SLEEP / WAKE	WET	POOP
		LEFT				
		RIGHT				
		L:				
		R:				
		L:				
		R:				
		L:				
		R:				
		L:				
		R:				
		L:				
		R:				
		L:				
		R:				
		L:				
		R:				
		L:				
		R:				
		L:				
		R:				
		L:				
		R:				
		L:				
		R:				

Notes & Milestones:

Baby's Eat, Sleep & Poop Daily Activity

DATE	TIME	MINUTES (Breastfeeding)	OUNCES (Bottle)	SLEEP WAKE	WET	POOP
		LEFT				
		RIGHT				
		L:				
		R:				
		L:				
		R:				
		L:				
		R:				
		L:				
		R:				
		L:				
		R:				
		L:				
		R:				
		L:				
		R:				
		L:				
		R:				
		L:				
		R:				
		L:				
		R:				
		L:				
		R:				
		L:				
		R:				

Notes & Milestones:

Baby's Eat, Sleep & Poop Daily Activity

DATE	TIME	MINUTES (Breastfeeding)	OUNCES (Bottle)	SLEEP WAKE	WET	POOP
		LEFT				
		RIGHT				
		L:				
		R:				
		L:				
		R:				
		L:				
		R:				
		L:				
		R:				
		L:				
		R:				
		L:				
		R:				
		L:				
		R:				
		L:				
		R:				
		L:				
		R:				
		L:				
		R:				
		L:				
		R:				
		L:				
		R:				
		L:				
		R:				

Notes & Milestones:

Baby's Eat, Sleep & Poop Daily Activity

DATE	TIME	MINUTES (Breastfeeding)	OUNCES (Bottle)	SLEEP / WAKE	WET	POOP
		LEFT:				
		RIGHT:				
		L:				
		R:				
		L:				
		R:				
		L:				
		R:				
		L:				
		R:				
		L:				
		R:				
		L:				
		R:				
		L:				
		R:				
		L:				
		R:				
		L:				
		R:				
		L:				
		R:				
		L:				
		R:				
		L:				
		R:				

Notes & Milestones:

Baby's Eat, Sleep & Poop Daily Activity

DATE	TIME	MINUTES (Breastfeeding)	OUNCES (Bottle)	SLEEP WAKE	WET	POOP
		LEFT				
		RIGHT				
		L:				
		R:				
		L:				
		R:				
		L:				
		R:				
		L:				
		R:				
		L:				
		R:				
		L:				
		R:				
		L:				
		R:				
		L:				
		R:				
		L:				
		R:				
		L:				
		R:				
		L:				
		R:				

Notes & Milestones:

Baby's Eat, Sleep & Poop Daily Activity

DATE	TIME	MINUTES (Breastfeeding)	OUNCES (Bottle)	SLEEP WAKE	WET	POOP
		LEFT				
		RIGHT				
		L:				
		R:				
		L:				
		R:				
		L:				
		R:				
		L:				
		R:				
		L:				
		R:				
		L:				
		R:				
		L:				
		R:				
		L:				
		R:				
		L:				
		R:				
		L:				
		R:				
		L:				
		R:				
		L:				

©2004-2020 SK Creative Agency Inc. All rights reserved. eatsleeppoop.com

Notes & Milestones:

Baby's Eat, Sleep & Poop Daily Activity

DATE	TIME	MINUTES (Breastfeeding)	OUNCES (Bottle)	SLEEP WAKE	WET	POOP
		LEFT				
		RIGHT				
		L:				
		R:				
		L:				
		R:				
		L:				
		R:				
		L:				
		R:				
		L:				
		R:				
		L:				
		R:				
		L:				
		R:				
		L:				
		R:				
		L:				
		R:				
		L:				
		R:				
		L:				
		R:				
		L:				
		R:				

©2004-2020 SK Creative Agency Inc. All rights reserved. earlysleeppppp.com

Notes & Milestones:

Baby's Eat, Sleep & Poop Daily Activity

DATE	TIME	MINUTES (Breastfeeding)	OUNCES (Bottle)	SLEEP / WAKE	WET	POOP
		LEFT				
		RIGHT				
		L:				
		R:				
		L:				
		R:				
		L:				
		R:				
		L:				
		R:				
		L:				
		R:				
		L:				
		R:				
		L:				
		R:				
		L:				
		R:				
		L:				
		R:				
		L:				
		R:				
		L:				
		R:				
		L:				
		R:				

©2004-2020 SK Creative Agency Inc. All rights reserved. eatsleeppoop.com

Notes & Milestones:

Baby's Eat, Sleep & Poop Daily Activity

DATE	TIME	MINUTES (Breastfeeding)	OUNCES (Bottle)	SLEEP / WAKE	WET	POOP
		LEFT				
		RIGHT				
		L:				
		R:				
		L:				
		R:				
		L:				
		R:				
		L:				
		R:				
		L:				
		R:				
		L:				
		R:				
		L:				
		R:				
		L:				
		R:				
		L:				
		R:				
		L:				
		R:				
		L:				
		R:				
		L:				
		R:				

©2004-2020 SK Creative Agency Inc. All rights reserved. eatsleeppoop.com

Notes & Milestones:

Baby's Eat, Sleep & Poop Daily Activity

DATE	TIME	MINUTES (Breastfeeding)	OUNCES (Bottle)	SLEEP WAKE	WET	POOP
		LEFT				
		RIGHT				
		L:				
		R:				
		L:				
		R:				
		L:				
		R:				
		L:				
		R:				
		L:				
		R:				
		L:				
		R:				
		L:				
		R:				
		L:				
		R:				
		L:				
		R:				
		L:				
		R:				
		L:				
		R:				
		L:				
		R:				

©2004-2020 SK Creative Agency Inc. All rights reserved. eatsleeppoop.com

Notes & Milestones:

Baby's Eat, Sleep & Poop Daily Activity

DATE	TIME	MINUTES (Breastfeeding)		OUNCES (Bottle)	SLEEP WAKE	WET	POOP
		LEFT					
		RIGHT					
		L:					
		R:					
		L:					
		R:					
		L:					
		R:					
		L:					
		R:					
		L:					
		R:					
		L:					
		R:					
		L:					
		R:					
		L:					
		R:					
		L:					
		R:					
		L:					
		R:					
		L:					
		R:					
		L:					
		R:					

©2004-2020 SK Creative Agency Inc. All rights reserved. eatsleeppoop.com

Notes & Milestones:

Baby's Eat, Sleep & Poop Daily Activity

DATE	TIME	MINUTES (Breastfeeding)		OUNCES (Bottle)	SLEEP / WAKE	WET	POOP
		LEFT					
		RIGHT					
		L:					
		R:					
		L:					
		R:					
		L:					
		R:					
		L:					
		R:					
		L:					
		R:					
		L:					
		R:					
		L:					
		R:					
		L:					
		R:					
		L:					
		R:					
		L:					
		R:					
		L:					
		R:					
		L:					
		R:					

Notes & Milestones:

Baby's Eat, Sleep & Poop Daily Activity

DATE	TIME	MINUTES (Breastfeeding)		OUNCES (Bottle)	SLEEP WAKE	WET	POOP
		LEFT:					
		RIGHT:					
		L:					
		R:					
		L:					
		R:					
		L:					
		R:					
		L:					
		R:					
		L:					
		R:					
		L:					
		R:					
		L:					
		R:					
		L:					
		R:					
		L:					
		R:					
		L:					
		R:					
		L:					
		R:					
		L:					
		R:					

©2004-2020 SK Creative Agency Inc. All rights reserved. eatsleepoop.com

Notes & Milestones:

Baby's Eat, Sleep & Poop Daily Activity

DATE	TIME	MINUTES (Breastfeeding)	OUNCES (Bottle)	SLEEP WAKE	WET	POOP
		LEFT				
		RIGHT				
		L:				
		R:				
		L:				
		R:				
		L:				
		R:				
		L:				
		R:				
		L:				
		R:				
		L:				
		R:				
		L:				
		R:				
		L:				
		R:				
		L:				
		R:				
		L:				
		R:				
		L:				
		R:				
		L:				
		R:				

©2004-2020 SK Creative Agency Inc. All rights reserved. eatsleepoopon.com

Notes & Milestones:

Baby's Eat, Sleep & Poop Daily Activity

DATE	TIME	MINUTES (Breastfeeding)	OUNCES (Bottle)	SLEEP WAKE	WET	POOP
		LEFT				
		RIGHT				
		L:				
		R:				
		L:				
		R:				
		L:				
		R:				
		L:				
		R:				
		L:				
		R:				
		L:				
		R:				
		L:				
		R:				
		L:				
		R:				
		L:				
		R:				
		L:				
		R:				
		L:				
		R:				
		L:				
		R:				

©2004-2020 SK Creative Agency Inc. All rights reserved. getsleepnnnnn.com

Notes & Milestones:

Baby's Eat, Sleep & Poop Daily Activity

DATE	TIME	MINUTES (Breastfeeding)	OUNCES (Bottle)	SLEEP WAKE	WET	POOP
		LEFT				
		RIGHT				
		L:				
		R:				
		L:				
		R:				
		L:				
		R:				
		L:				
		R:				
		L:				
		R:				
		L:				
		R:				
		L:				
		R:				
		L:				
		R:				
		L:				
		R:				
		L:				
		R:				
		L:				
		R:				
		L:				
		R:				

©2004-2020 SK Creative Agency Inc. All rights reserved. eatsleeppoop.com

Notes & Milestones:

Baby's Eat, Sleep & Poop Daily Activity

DATE	TIME	MINUTES (Breastfeeding)	OUNCES (Bottle)	SLEEP WAKE	WET	POOP
		LEFT				
		RIGHT				
		L:				
		R:				
		L:				
		R:				
		L:				
		R:				
		L:				
		R:				
		L:				
		R:				
		L:				
		R:				
		L:				
		R:				
		L:				
		R:				
		L:				
		R:				
		L:				
		R:				
		L:				
		R:				
		L:				
		R:				

©2004-2020 SK Creative Agency Inc. All rights reserved. eatsleeppoop.com

Notes & Milestones:

Baby's Eat, Sleep & Poop Daily Activity

DATE	TIME	MINUTES (Breastfeeding)	OUNCES (Bottle)	SLEEP / WAKE	WET	POOP
		LEFT:				
		RIGHT:				
		L:				
		R:				
		L:				
		R:				
		L:				
		R:				
		L:				
		R:				
		L:				
		R:				
		L:				
		R:				
		L:				
		R:				
		L:				
		R:				
		L:				
		R:				
		L:				
		R:				
		L:				
		R:				
		L:				
		R:				

©2004-2020 SK Creative Agency Inc. All rights reserved. eatsleeppoop.com

Notes & Milestones:

Baby's Eat, Sleep & Poop Daily Activity

DATE	TIME	MINUTES (Breastfeeding)	OUNCES (Bottle)	SLEEP / WAKE	WET	POOP
		LEFT				
		RIGHT				
		L:				
		R:				
		L:				
		R:				
		L:				
		R:				
		L:				
		R:				
		L:				
		R:				
		L:				
		R:				
		L:				
		R:				
		L:				
		R:				
		L:				
		R:				
		L:				
		R:				
		L:				
		R:				
		L:				
		R:				

©2004-2020 SK Creative Agency Inc. All rights reserved. eatsleeppoop.com

Notes & Milestones:

Baby's Eat, Sleep & Poop Daily Activity

DATE	TIME	MINUTES (Breastfeeding)		OUNCES (Bottle)	SLEEP WAKE	WET	POOP
		LEFT					
		RIGHT					
		L:					
		R:					
		L:					
		R:					
		L:					
		R:					
		L:					
		R:					
		L:					
		R:					
		L:					
		R:					
		L:					
		R:					
		L:					
		R:					
		L:					
		R:					
		L:					
		R:					
		L:					
		R:					
		L:					
		R:					

©2004-2020 SK Creative Agency Inc. All rights reserved. eatsleeppoop.com

Notes & Milestones:

Baby's Eat, Sleep & Poop Daily Activity

DATE	TIME	MINUTES (Breastfeeding)	OUNCES (Bottle)	SLEEP / WAKE	WET	POOP
		LEFT				
		RIGHT				
		L:				
		R:				
		L:				
		R:				
		L:				
		R:				
		L:				
		R:				
		L:				
		R:				
		L:				
		R:				
		L:				
		R:				
		L:				
		R:				
		L:				
		R:				
		L:				
		R:				
		L:				
		R:				
		L:				
		R:				

©2004-2020 SK Creative Agency Inc. All rights reserved. eatsleeppoop.com

Notes & Milestones:

Baby's Eat, Sleep & Poop Daily Activity

DATE	TIME	MINUTES (Breastfeeding)	OUNCES (Bottle)	SLEEP / WAKE	WET	POOP
		LEFT				
		RIGHT				
		L:				
		R:				
		L:				
		R:				
		L:				
		R:				
		L:				
		R:				
		L:				
		R:				
		L:				
		R:				
		L:				
		R:				
		L:				
		R:				
		L:				
		R:				
		L:				
		R:				
		L:				
		R:				
		L:				
		R:				

©2004-2020 SK Creative Agency Inc. All rights reserved. eatsleeppoop.com

Notes & Milestones:

Baby's Eat, Sleep & Poop Daily Activity

DATE	TIME	MINUTES (Breastfeeding)	OUNCES (Bottle)	SLEEP WAKE	WET	POOP
		LEFT				
		RIGHT				
		L:				
		R:				
		L:				
		R:				
		L:				
		R:				
		L:				
		R:				
		L:				
		R:				
		L:				
		R:				
		L:				
		R:				
		L:				
		R:				
		L:				
		R:				
		L:				
		R:				
		L:				
		R:				
		L:				
		R:				

©2004-2020 SK Creative Agency Inc. All rights reserved. eatsleeppoop.com

Notes & Milestones:

Baby's Eat, Sleep & Poop Daily Activity

DATE	TIME	MINUTES (Breastfeeding)	OUNCES (Bottle)	SLEEP WAKE	WET	POOP
		LEFT				
		RIGHT				
		L:				
		R:				
		L:				
		R:				
		L:				
		R:				
		L:				
		R:				
		L:				
		R:				
		L:				
		R:				
		L:				
		R:				
		L:				
		R:				
		L:				
		R:				
		L:				
		R:				
		L:				
		R:				
		L:				
		R:				

Notes & Milestones:

Baby's Eat, Sleep & Poop Daily Activity

DATE	TIME	MINUTES (Breastfeeding)	OUNCES (Bottle)	SLEEP / WAKE	WET	POOP
		LEFT				
		RIGHT				
		L:				
		R:				
		L:				
		R:				
		L:				
		R:				
		L:				
		R:				
		L: .				
		R:				
		L:				
		R:				
		L:				
		R:				
		L:				
		R:				
		L:				
		R:				
		L:				
		R:				
		L:				
		R:				
		L:				
		R:				

©2004-2020 SK Creative Agency Inc. All rights reserved. eatsleeppooop.com

Notes & Milestones:

Baby's Eat, Sleep & Poop Daily Activity

DATE	TIME	MINUTES (Breastfeeding)	OUNCES (Bottle)	SLEEP WAKE	WET	POOP
		LEFT				
		RIGHT				
		L:				
		R:				
		L:				
		R:				
		L:				
		R:				
		L:				
		R:				
		L:				
		R:				
		L:				
		R:				
		L:				
		R:				
		L:				
		R:				
		L:				
		R:				
		L:				
		R:				
		L:				
		R:				
		L:				
		R:				

Notes & Milestones:

Baby's Eat, Sleep & Poop Daily Activity

DATE	TIME	MINUTES (Breastfeeding)	OUNCES (Bottle)	SLEEP WAKE	WET	POOP
		LEFT				
		RIGHT				
		L:				
		R:				
		L:				
		R:				
		L:				
		R:				
		L:				
		R:				
		L:				
		R:				
		L:				
		R:				
		L:				
		R:				
		L:				
		R:				
		L:				
		R:				
		L:				
		R:				
		L:				
		R:				
		L:				
		R:				

Notes & Milestones:

Baby's Eat, Sleep & Poop Daily Activity

DATE	TIME	MINUTES (Breastfeeding)	OUNCES (Bottle)	SLEEP WAKE	WET	POOP
		LEFT				
		RIGHT				
		L:				
		R:				
		L:				
		R:				
		L:				
		R:				
		L:				
		R:				
		L:				
		R:				
		L:				
		R:				
		L:				
		R:				
		L:				
		R:				
		L:				
		R:				
		L:				
		R:				
		L:				
		R:				
		L:				
		R:				

Notes & Milestones:

Baby's Eat, Sleep & Poop Daily Activity

DATE	TIME	MINUTES (Breastfeeding)	OUNCES (Bottle)	SLEEP WAKE	WET	POOP
		LEFT				
		RIGHT				
		L:				
		R:				
		L:				
		R:				
		L:				
		R:				
		L:				
		R:				
		L:				
		R:				
		L:				
		R:				
		L:				
		R:				
		L:				
		R:				
		L:				
		R:				
		L:				
		R:				
		L:				
		R:				
		L:				
		R:				

©2004-2020 SK Creative Agency Inc. All rights reserved. eatsleeppoop.com

Notes & Milestones:

Baby's Eat, Sleep & Poop Daily Activity

DATE	TIME	MINUTES (Breastfeeding)	OUNCES (Bottle)	SLEEP / WAKE	WET	POOP
		LEFT				
		RIGHT				
		L:				
		R:				
		L:				
		R:				
		L:				
		R:				
		L:				
		R:				
		L:				
		R:				
		L:				
		R:				
		L:				
		R:				
		L:				
		R:				
		L:				
		R:				
		L:				
		R:				
		L:				
		R:				
		L:				
		R:				

©2004-2020 SK Creative Agency Inc. All rights reserved. eatsleepnpoop.com

Notes & Milestones:

Baby's Eat, Sleep & Poop Daily Activity

DATE	TIME	MINUTES (Breastfeeding)	OUNCES (Bottle)	SLEEP WAKE	WET	POOP
		LEFT				
		RIGHT				
		L:				
		R:				
		L:				
		R:				
		L:				
		R:				
		L:				
		R:				
		L:				
		R:				
		L:				
		R:				
		L:				
		R:				
		L:				
		R:				
		L:				
		R:				
		L:				
		R:				
		L:				
		R:				
		L:				
		R:				

©2004-2020 SK Creative Agency Inc. All rights reserved.

Notes & Milestones:

Baby's Eat, Sleep & Poop Daily Activity

DATE	TIME	MINUTES (Breastfeeding)		OUNCES (Bottle)	SLEEP WAKE	WET	POOP
		LEFT					
		RIGHT					
		L:					
		R:					
		L:					
		R:					
		L:					
		R:					
		L:					
		R:					
		L:					
		R:					
		L:					
		R:					
		L:					
		R:					
		L:					
		R:					
		L:					
		R:					
		L:					
		R:					
		L:					
		R:					
		L:					
		R:					

©2004-2020 SK Creative Agency Inc. All rights reserved. eatsleeppoop.com

Notes & Milestones:

Baby's Eat, Sleep & Poop Daily Activity

DATE	TIME	MINUTES (Breastfeeding)	OUNCES (Bottle)	SLEEP WAKE	WET	POOP
		LEFT				
		RIGHT				
		L:				
		R:				
		L:				
		R:				
		L:				
		R:				
		L:				
		R:				
		L:				
		R:				
		L:				
		R:				
		L:				
		R:				
		L:				
		R:				
		L:				
		R:				
		L:				
		R:				
		L:				
		R:				
		L:				
		R:				

©2004-2020 SK Creative Agency Inc. All rights reserved. eatsleeppoop.com

Notes & Milestones:

Baby's Eat, Sleep & Poop Daily Activity

DATE	TIME	MINUTES (Breastfeeding)	OUNCES (Bottle)	SLEEP WAKE	WET	POOP
		LEFT				
		RIGHT				
		L:				
		R:				
		L:				
		R:				
		L:				
		R:				
		L:				
		R:				
		L:				
		R:				
		L:				
		R:				
		L:				
		R:				
		L:				
		R:				
		L:				
		R:				
		L:				
		R:				
		L:				
		R:				
		L:				
		R:				

©2004-2020 SK Creative Agency Inc. All rights reserved. eatsleeppoop.com

Notes & Milestones:

Baby's Eat, Sleep & Poop Daily Activity

DATE	TIME	MINUTES (Breastfeeding)	OUNCES (Bottle)	SLEEP WAKE	WET	POOP
		LEFT				
		RIGHT				
		L:				
		R:				
		L:				
		R:				
		L:				
		R:				
		L:				
		R:				
		L:				
		R:				
		L:				
		R:				
		L:				
		R:				
		L:				
		R:				
		L:				
		R:				
		L:				
		R:				
		L:				
		R:				
		L:				
		R:				

Notes & Milestones:

Baby's Eat, Sleep & Poop Daily Activity

DATE	TIME	MINUTES (Breastfeeding)	OUNCES (Bottle)	SLEEP / WAKE	WET	POOP
		LEFT				
		RIGHT				
		L:				
		R:				
		L:				
		R:				
		L:				
		R:				
		L:				
		R:				
		L:				
		R:				
		L:				
		R:				
		L:				
		R:				
		L:				
		R:				
		L:				
		R:				
		L:				
		R:				
		L:				
		R:				
		L:				
		R:				

Notes & Milestones:

Baby's Eat, Sleep & Poop Daily Activity

DATE	TIME	MINUTES (Breastfeeding)	OUNCES (Bottle)	SLEEP WAKE	WET	POOP
		LEFT				
		RIGHT				
		L:				
		R:				
		L:				
		R:				
		L:				
		R:				
		L:				
		R:				
		L:				
		R:				
		L:				
		R:				
		L:				
		R:				
		L:				
		R:				
		L:				
		R:				
		L:				
		R:				
		L:				
		R:				
		L:				
		R:				

Notes & Milestones:

Baby's Eat, Sleep & Poop Daily Activity

DATE	TIME	MINUTES (Breastfeeding)	OUNCES (Bottle)	SLEEP WAKE	WET	POOP
		LEFT				
		RIGHT				
		L:				
		R:				
		L:				
		R:				
		L:				
		R:				
		L:				
		R:				
		L:				
		R:				
		L:				
		R:				
		L:				
		R:				
		L:				
		R:				
		L:				
		R:				
		L:				
		R:				
		L:				
		R:				

Notes & Milestones:

Baby's Eat, Sleep & Poop Daily Activity

DATE	TIME	MINUTES (Breastfeeding)	OUNCES (Bottle)	SLEEP WAKE	WET	POOP
		LEFT:				
		RIGHT:				
		L:				
		R:				
		L:				
		R:				
		L:				
		R:				
		L:				
		R:				
		L:				
		R:				
		L:				
		R:				
		L:				
		R:				
		L:				
		R:				
		L:				
		R:				
		L:				
		R:				
		L:				
		R:				
		L:				
		R:				

Notes & Milestones:

Baby's Eat, Sleep & Poop Daily Activity

DATE	TIME	MINUTES (Breastfeeding)	OUNCES (Bottle)	SLEEP / WAKE	WET	POOP
		LEFT:				
		RIGHT:				
		L:				
		R:				
		L:				
		R:				
		L:				
		R:				
		L:				
		R:				
		L:				
		R:				
		L:				
		R:				
		L:				
		R:				
		L:				
		R:				
		L:				
		R:				
		L:				
		R:				
		L:				
		R:				
		L:				
		R:				

Notes & Milestones:

Baby's Eat, Sleep & Poop Daily Activity

DATE	TIME	MINUTES (Breastfeeding)	OUNCES (Bottle)	SLEEP WAKE	WET	POOP
		LEFT				
		RIGHT				
		L:				
		R:				
		L:				
		R:				
		L:				
		R:				
		L:				
		R:				
		L:				
		R:				
		L:				
		R:				
		L:				
		R:				
		L:				
		R:				
		L:				
		R:				
		L:				
		R:				
		L:				
		R:				
		L:				
		R:				

©2004-2020 SK Creative Agency Inc. All rights reserved. earlsleeppoop.com

Notes & Milestones:

Baby's Eat, Sleep & Poop Daily Activity

DATE	TIME	MINUTES (Breastfeeding)	OUNCES (Bottle)	SLEEP WAKE	WET	POOP
		LEFT				
		RIGHT				
		L:				
		R:				
		L:				
		R:				
		L:				
		R:				
		L:				
		R:				
		L:				
		R:				
		L:				
		R:				
		L:				
		R:				
		L:				
		R:				
		L:				
		R:				
		L:				
		R:				
		L:				
		R:				
		L:				
		R:				

©2004-2020 SK Creative Agency Inc. All rights reserved. eatsleeppoop.com

Notes & Milestones:

Baby's Eat, Sleep & Poop Daily Activity

DATE	TIME	MINUTES (Breastfeeding)	OUNCES (Bottle)	SLEEP WAKE	WET	POOP
		LEFT				
		RIGHT				
		L:				
		R:				
		L:				
		R:				
		L:				
		R:				
		L:				
		R:				
		L:				
		R:				
		L:				
		R:				
		L:				
		R:				
		L:				
		R:				
		L:				
		R:				
		L:				
		R:				
		L:				
		R:				
		L:				
		R:				

Notes & Milestones:

Baby's Eat, Sleep & Poop Daily Activity

DATE	TIME	MINUTES (Breastfeeding)	OUNCES (Bottle)	SLEEP WAKE	WET	POOP
		LEFT:				
		RIGHT:				
		L:				
		R:				
		L:				
		R:				
		L:				
		R:				
		L:				
		R:				
		L:				
		R:				
		L:				
		R:				
		L:				
		R:				
		L:				
		R:				
		L:				
		R:				
		L:				
		R:				
		L:				
		R:				
		L:				
		R:				

Notes & Milestones:

Baby's Eat, Sleep & Poop Daily Activity

DATE	TIME	MINUTES (Breastfeeding)	OUNCES (Bottle)	SLEEP / WAKE	WET	POOP
		LEFT				
		RIGHT				
		L:				
		R:				
		L:				
		R:				
		L:				
		R:				
		L:				
		R:				
		L:				
		R:				
		L:				
		R:				
		L:				
		R:				
		L:				
		R:				
		L:				
		R:				
		L:				
		R:				
		L:				
		R:				

Notes & Milestones:

Baby's Eat, Sleep & Poop Daily Activity

DATE	TIME	MINUTES (Breastfeeding)	OUNCES (Bottle)	SLEEP / WAKE	WET	POOP
		LEFT				
		RIGHT				
		L:				
		R:				
		L:				
		R:				
		L:				
		R:				
		L:				
		R:				
		L:				
		R:				
		L:				
		R:				
		L:				
		R:				
		L:				
		R:				
		L:				
		R:				
		L:				
		R:				
		L:				
		R:				
		L:				
		R:				

©2004-2020 SK Creative Agency Inc. All rights reserved. eatsleeppoop.com

Notes & Milestones:

Baby's Eat, Sleep & Poop Daily Activity

DATE	TIME	MINUTES (Breastfeeding)	OUNCES (Bottle)	SLEEP WAKE	WET	POOP
		LEFT				
		RIGHT				
		L:				
		R:				
		L:				
		R:				
		L:				
		R:				
		L:				
		R:				
		L:				
		R:				
		L:				
		R:				
		L:				
		R:				
		L:				
		R:				
		L:				
		R:				
		L:				
		R:				
		L:				
		R:				
		L:				
		R:				

Notes & Milestones:

Baby's Eat, Sleep & Poop Daily Activity

DATE	TIME	MINUTES (Breastfeeding)	OUNCES (Bottle)	SLEEP WAKE	WET	POOP
		LEFT:				
		RIGHT:				
		L:				
		R:				
		L:				
		R:				
		L:				
		R:				
		L:				
		R:				
		L:				
		R:				
		L:				
		R:				
		L:				
		R:				
		L:				
		R:				
		L:				
		R:				
		L:				
		R:				
		L:				
		R:				
		L:				
		R:				

©2004-2020 SK Creative Agency Inc. All rights reserved. eatsleeppoop.com

Notes & Milestones:

Baby's Eat, Sleep & Poop Daily Activity

DATE	TIME	MINUTES (Breastfeeding)	OUNCES (Bottle)	SLEEP WAKE	WET	POOP
		LEFT				
		RIGHT				
		L:				
		R:				
		L:				
		R:				
		L:				
		R:				
		L:				
		R:				
		L:				
		R:				
		L:				
		R:				
		L:				
		R:				
		L:				
		R:				
		L:				
		R:				
		L:				
		R:				
		L:				
		R:				
		L:				
		R:				

Notes & Milestones:

Baby's Eat, Sleep & Poop Daily Activity

DATE	TIME	MINUTES (Breastfeeding)	OUNCES (Bottle)	SLEEP WAKE	WET	POOP
		LEFT				
		RIGHT				
		L:				
		R:				
		L:				
		R:				
		L:				
		R:				
		L:				
		R:				
		L:				
		R:				
		L:				
		R:				
		L:				
		R:				
		L:				
		R:				
		L:				
		R:				
		L:				
		R:				
		L:				
		R:				
		L:				
		R:				

Notes & Milestones:

Baby's Eat, Sleep & Poop Daily Activity

DATE	TIME	MINUTES (Breastfeeding)	OUNCES (Bottle)	SLEEP WAKE	WET	POOP
		LEFT:				
		RIGHT:				
		L:				
		R:				
		L:				
		R:				
		L:				
		R:				
		L:				
		R:				
		L:				
		R:				
		L:				
		R:				
		L:				
		R:				
		L:				
		R:				
		L:				
		R:				
		L:				
		R:				
		L:				
		R:				
		L:				
		R:				

Notes & Milestones:

Baby's Eat, Sleep & Poop Daily Activity

DATE	TIME	MINUTES (Breastfeeding)	OUNCES (Bottle)	SLEEP WAKE	WET	POOP
		LEFT				
		RIGHT				
		L:				
		R:				
		L:				
		R:				
		L:				
		R:				
		L:				
		R:				
		L:				
		R:				
		L:				
		R:				
		L:				
		R:				
		L:				
		R:				
		L:				
		R:				
		L:				
		R:				
		L:				
		R:				
		L:				
		R:				

Notes & Milestones:

Baby's Eat, Sleep & Poop Daily Activity

DATE	TIME	MINUTES (Breastfeeding)	OUNCES (Bottle)	SLEEP WAKE	WET	POOP
		LEFT				
		RIGHT				
		L:				
		R:				
		L:				
		R:				
		L:				
		R:				
		L:				
		R:				
		L:				
		R:				
		L:				
		R:				
		L:				
		R:				
		L:				
		R:				
		L:				
		R:				
		L:				
		R:				
		L:				
		R:				
		L:				
		R:				

Notes & Milestones:

Baby's Eat, Sleep & Poop Daily Activity

DATE	TIME	MINUTES (Breastfeeding)	OUNCES (Bottle)	SLEEP WAKE	WET	POOP
		LEFT				
		RIGHT				
		L:				
		R:				
		L:				
		R:				
		L:				
		R:				
		L:				
		R:				
		L:				
		R:				
		L:				
		R:				
		L:				
		R:				
		L:				
		R:				
		L:				
		R:				
		L:				
		R:				
		L:				
		R:				
		L:				
		R:				

©2004-2020 SK Creative Agency Inc. All rights reserved.

Notes & Milestones:

Baby's Eat, Sleep & Poop Daily Activity

DATE	TIME	MINUTES (Breastfeeding)	OUNCES (Bottle)	SLEEP / WAKE	WET	POOP
		LEFT				
		RIGHT				
		L:				
		R:				
		L:				
		R:				
		L:				
		R:				
		L:				
		R:				
		L:				
		R:				
		L:				
		R:				
		L:				
		R:				
		L:				
		R:				
		L:				
		R:				
		L:				
		R:				
		L:				
		R:				
		L:				
		R:				

Notes & Milestones: